MY OWN PCP

(Personal Care Provider)

WORKBOOK

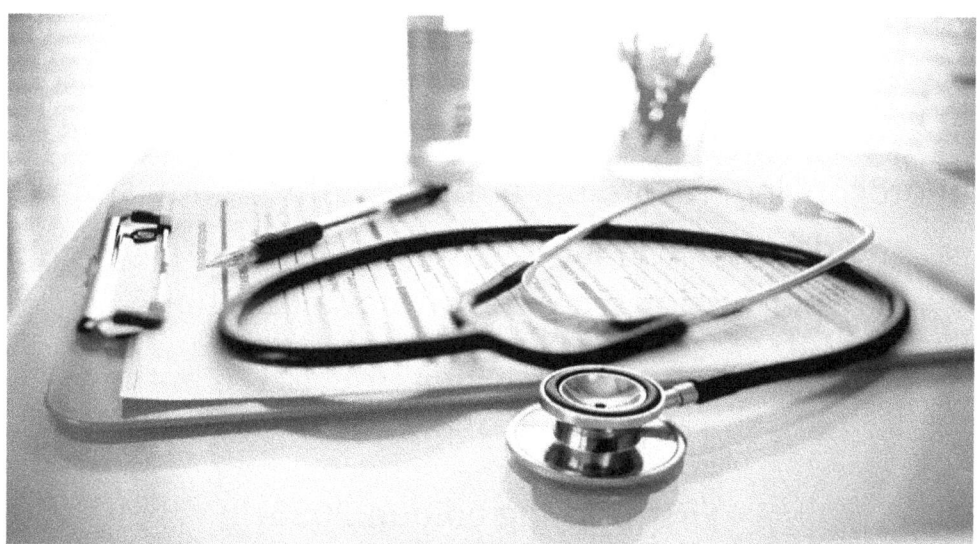

Unlocking your Health potential for Life

Copyright © 2025 Danielle Shears

ALL RIGHTS RESERVED. This book contains material protected under International and Federal Copyright Laws and Treaties. Any unauthorized reprint or use of this material is prohibited. No part of this book may be reproduced or transmitted in any form or by any means, electronic or mechanical, including photocopying, recording, or by any information storage and retrieval system without express written permission from the author/publisher.

Printed by Prize Publishing House, LLC in the United States of America.

First printing edition 2025.

Prize Publishing House

P.O. Box 9856, Chesapeake, VA 23321

www.PrizePublishingHouse.com

ISBN (Paperback): 979-8-9925617-6-0

This Book Belongs to:

Name: _____

_____

Phone: _____

_____

Email: _____

_____

Disclaimer

The information and resources provided in this workbook and calendar are intended for educational and informational purposes only.

While this workbook is designed to help you take charge of your health, it is not a substitute for professional medical advice, diagnosis, or treatment. Always seek the advice of your physician or other qualified health providers with any questions you may have regarding your medical condition or treatment.

While the intent of this workbook is to encourage you to take charge of your health, never disregard professional medical advice or delay in seeking it because of something you have read in this workbook. Rather, use this information to help guide conversations with your healthcare provider.

Your health and well-being are important, and it is essential to consult with your healthcare provider before making significant changes to your diet, exercise, or health management plans.

By using this workbook, you acknowledge and agree that you are solely responsible for your health decisions and that the author shall not be liable for any actions taken based on the information provided herein.

Introduction

Welcome to your journey toward better health and well-being! This workbook is designed to empower you to take charge of your health through practical strategies, mindful practices, and effective tracking tools. Whether you are looking to enhance your overall wellness, improve specific health markers, or simply cultivate a more balanced lifestyle, this workbook will serve as your trusted companion every step of the way.

Section One: Mindfulness, goal setting and Self-Care

In the first section, you'll discover a wealth of tips and techniques focused on mindfulness, self-love, and stress reduction. You'll learn how to incorporate mindfulness practices into your daily routine, fostering a deeper connection with yourself and your emotions. We'll explore the importance of self-love and how it can positively impact your mental and physical health. Additionally, you'll find valuable strategies for improving your sleep quality and sample exercises designed to boost your mood and energy levels.

Section Two: Health Toolkit

The second section offers a comprehensive health toolkit, including essential information on lab values and tracking sheets for monitoring key health indicators such as blood pressure, diabetes, and other health concerns. This toolkit will empower you to take an active role in your health management, enabling you to have informed discussions with your healthcare provider and make data-driven decisions.

Section Three: Working Calendar

Finally, the third section features a working calendar with weekly sheets that will help you track your daily and weekly progress.

This structured approach allows you to set goals, monitor your achievements, and celebrate your successes. By regularly assessing your progress, you can make informed adjustments to your health journey, ensuring that you stay on track and motivated.

As you embark on this journey, remember that taking charge of your health is a personal and unique experience. Use this workbook as a resource to guide you, inspire you, and support yourself in your quest for a healthier, happier you.

Let's get started!

Table of Contents

Section One: Mindfulness Techniques, Goal Settings, and Self-Care

1. Motivational Quotes
2. Designing a Personal Mission Statement
3. Mindfulness Technique
4. Tips for a Better Night's Sleep
5. Stress Relieving Techniques
6. MSRP Evaluation
7. Morning Five/Night Cap Three
8. Sample HITT Workouts
9. Goal Setting
10. Build Your Team
11. Self-Reflection
12. Areas of Opportunity
13. QR Code

Section Two: Health Toolkit

1. Blood Glucose Tracker
2. Blood Pressure Tracker
3. Exercise Tracker
4. Lab Tracker
5. Symptom Tracker
6. Weight Tracker
7. Family Medical History
8. My Medical History
9. I am Monitoring
10. Medication Tracker
11. Physician Record
12. Advance Directives
13. Test Results
14. Action Plan

Section Three: Calendar

PLEASE NOTE: Click the QR code to gain further instruction and insight into the flow of this workbook. I'm looking forward to working with you to achieve your goals:

Section 1

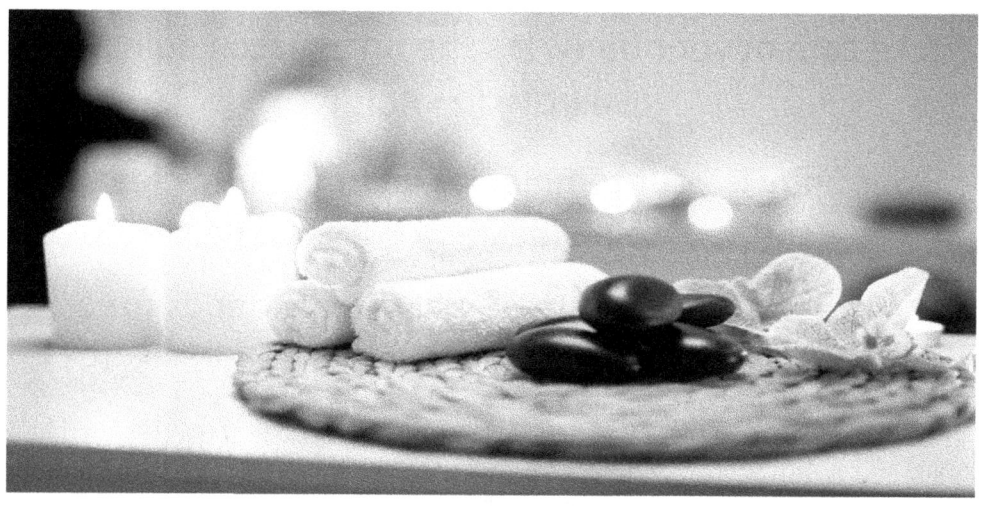

Mindfulness, Goal Setting, and Self-Care

Motivational Quotes

"Your body is your most valuable asset. Take care of it, and it will take care of you." – Unknown

"Take care of your body. It's the only place you have to live in." - Jim Rohn

"Your body is your temple. Keep it pure and clean for the soul to reside in." - B.K.S. Iyengar

"Invest in your health, it will pay dividends for a lifetime." – Unknown

"The greatest wealth is health."– Virgil

"Your body is a reflection of how you treat it. Take care of it, and it will take care of you."

– Unknown

"Your body is your most priceless possession. Take care of it." - Jack LaLanne

"Your body is your vehicle for success. Take care of it and it will take you wherever you want to go"

– Unknown

"Your body is your home. Treat it with love and it will always be a safe haven." – Unknown

"Progress is Impossible without change and those who cannot change their minds cannot change anything"

George Bernard Shaw

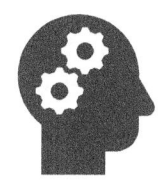 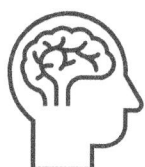 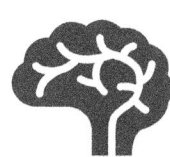

Designing a personal mission statement involves reflecting on your values, passions, and goals in order to define your purpose and guide your actions. Here is a step-by-step guide to help you create a personal mission statement.

1. Self-Reflection

Take some time for self-reflection and consider what is truly important to you. Think about your values, interests, strengths, and what brings you fulfillment. Reflect on your passions, aspirations, and what you want to achieve in different areas of your life.

2. Identify Core Values

Determine the core values that guide your life. These are the principles and beliefs that are most important to you. Consider what qualities and virtues you want to uphold and prioritize in your actions and decisions.

3. Define Your Purpose

Clarify your purpose or the overarching reason for your existence. What is the unique contribution you want to make in the world? Think about how you can align your values, passions, and skills to serve a greater purpose or make a positive impact on others.

4. Set Goals and Objectives

Identify specific goals and objectives that you want to achieve in different areas of your life, such as career, relationships, personal growth, health, and community involvement. These goals should be aligned with your purpose and values.

5. Craft a Personal Mission Statement

Use the insights gained from self-reflection, values, purpose, and goals to create a personal mission statement. It should be a concise, powerful, and inspiring statement that captures the essence of who you are and what you want to achieve.

6. Prioritize and Align

Use your mission statement as a guide to prioritize your actions, decisions, and commitments. Ensure that your daily activities align with your mission statement and contribute to your overall goals and purpose.

7. Review and Revise

Regularly review your personal mission statement and assess if it still resonates with you and reflects your current aspirations and values. Revise and update it as needed to stay aligned with your evolving journey.

8. Live Your Mission

Integrate your mission statement into your daily life. Let it be a source of inspiration and motivation, guiding your choices and actions. Continuously strive to live in alignment with your mission and make choices that move you closer to your goals and purpose.

My Personal Mission Statement

_____

_____

_____

_____

_____

_____

_____

_____

_____

_____

Mindfulness Techniques

1.

Start with short sessions:

Begin by setting aside a few minutes each day to practice mindfulness. Gradually increase the duration as you become more comfortable.

2.

Focus on the present moment:

Pay attention to your current experience without judgment. Notice your thoughts, emotions, bodily sensations, and the environment around you.

3.

Practice deep breathing:

Take slow, deep breaths, focusing on the sensation of the breath entering and leaving your body. This helps anchor your attention to the present moment.

4.

Engage in mindful activities:

Incorporate mindfulness into daily activities such as eating, walking, or even washing dishes. Pay attention to the sensations, smells, tastes, and sounds associated with these activities.

5.

Observe your thoughts:

Instead of getting caught up in your thoughts, try observing them without judgment. Notice them as passing mental events and gently redirect your attention back to the present moment.

6.

Practice body scan awareness:

Lie down or sit comfortably and systematically focus your attention on different parts of your body, starting from your toes and moving up to your head. Appreciate any sensations or tension and allow them to be released.

7.

Build a team/Get accountability:

Consider asking someone to join you in practicing C mindfulness to help you stay motivated and on track. This can provide support, guidance, and accountability.

Remember, mindfulness is a skill that improves with practice. Be patient and kind to yourself as you develop this habit.

8 Tips for a Better Night's Sleep

1. SLEEP SCHEDULE

Have a regular sleep schedule. Meaning: go to bed around the same time every evening and get up around the same time every morning.

2. DIET

Don't eat too close to bedtime. Make sure that your last meal is at least 2 hours before you go to bed. Watch your caffeine intake. Caffeine can throw off your natural sleep rhythm if consumed too close to bedtime. Avoid alcohol, caffeine, and marijuana. Increase fiber: chia seeds are good. Decaffeinated chamomile tea is okay.

3. ENVIRONMENT

Be in Be intentional about the lighting and temperature in your room. You want it to be very dark! Try to sleep with blackout curtains so that the light will not disturb your sleep. Your core body temperature decreases at night, so you can turn down the temperature as low as 65°F. This will also make you fall asleep faster.

4. TECHNOLOGY

Eliminate cell phones and laptops close to bedtime. The blue light from the screen can interfere with a person's circadian rhythm. Keep your TV and your cell phone turned off at night or have them in a different room from your bedroom.

5. EPSOM SALT BATH

This can flush out toxins due to its ability to dilate the blood vessels near the skin.

6. GO TO BED EARLIER

The later you go to bed the more you interfere with the pattern of how your cortisol levels flow.

7. PROGRESSIVE MUSCLE RELAXATION

Progressive muscle relaxation exercises involve tensing and then relaxing specific muscle groups in your body. The purpose is to help you become more aware of the difference between muscle tension and relaxation, and to promote a state of deep relaxation throughout your body. During progressive muscle relaxation, you typically start by tensing a specific muscle group, such as your fists, arms, or shoulders, for a few seconds. Then, you release the tension and focus on the sensation of relaxation in that muscle group. This process is repeated for different muscle groups throughout your body, allowing you to progressively relax and release tension from head to toe.

These exercises can help reduce muscle tension, relieve stress, promote better sleep, and improve overall physical and mental relaxation. They can be particularly beneficial for individuals who experience chronic muscle tension or anxiety.

8. INCREASE MAGNESIUM

Magnesium glycinate or Magnesium citrate

Stress Relieving Techniques

1. Lower your cortisol levels:

Mix to make your favorite combination!

a. Vitamin C: fresh lemon/lime juice, fresh orange juice, vitamin C powder

b. Potassium: aloe vera, coconut water, electrolyte powder

c. Sodium: sea salt, electrolyte powder, coconut milk, collagen powder

2. Boxed or square breathing: Boxed breathing is a technique in which you make a "box" with your breath.

Here is how to do it:

1. Inhale through your nose for four seconds
2. Hold for four seconds
3. Exhale through the nose or mouth for four seconds
4. Repeat steps 1-3 for a total time of 60 seconds

OR

Paced breathing:

Here is how to do it:

1. Inhale through your nose for five seconds
2. Once the lungs are full, exhale through the nose or mouth for five seconds
3. Repeat steps 1 and 2 for a total time of 60 seconds

3. Epsom salt bath:

Simple version:

1 cup of Epsom salt in warm bath water. Soak for 20 minutes.

Max salt detox bath:

1/4 cup sea salt/Himalayan salt

1/4 cup Epsom salt

1/4 cup baking soda

1/3 cup apple cider vinegar 10 drops of your favorite essential oil (ex. lavender) Soak for 20 minutes.

Note: Be careful when getting out of the tub as a change in blood flow and detox may cause lightheadedness.

MSRP Evaluation

Start by rating yourself on a scale from 1-100 in each of the four categories below: Mindset, Self-Discipline, Resilience, Perseverance. (This is your **self-evaluation score, total MSRP**). Then answer the questions on the next page and add up the corresponding number value (This is the **question total**). Finally, tally your score to determine the likelihood of you reaching and maintaining your goals for life.

Mindset

Refers to a person's established set of attitudes, beliefs and thoughts that shape their perception and interpretation of the world. **On a scale from 1-100 how would you rate yourself?** _

Note: Mindset plays a crucial role in determining one's behavior, motivation, resilience, and overall success in various aspects of life.

Self-Discipline

Refers to the ability to control one's impulses, emotions, and behaviors to achieve specific goals or adhere to certain standards. Involves making conscious choices and taking actions that align with one's long-term objectives even in the face of distraction, temptations, or difficulties. **On a scale from 1-100 how would you rate yourself?** ___

Note: Considered a valuable trait as it enables individuals to overcome obstacles, stay committed to their goals and achieve personal or professional success.

Resilience

Refers to the ability to bounce back, adapt, and recover from adversity, challenges, or setbacks. The capacity to withstand and navigate through difficult or stressful situations, while maintaining a positive mindset and emotional well-being. **On a scale from 1-100 how would you rate yourself? ___**

Note: Developing resilience is important for personal growth, mental health, and overall, well-being as it helps individuals to navigate life's ups and downs with greater ease and adaptability.

Perseverance

Persistence in doing something despite difficulty or delay in achieving success. The quality of persisting in a task or goal despite facing challenges, obstacles, or setbacks. The ability to keep going, to stay committed, and to maintain a positive attitude even in the face of adversity. **On a scale from 1-100 how would you rate yourself? ___**

Note: Having perseverance is an essential trait for achieving success in any area of life. It is what allows individuals to overcome difficulties, learn from failures, and ultimately reach their desired outcomes.

Total of M + S + R + P = _____

MSRP Questionnaire

Add a checkmark next to any of the statements that describe you. When you're done, add the number values (each is either -5 or -10) that correspond to each statement, to come up with the total at the bottom.

____   Your initial approach to a situation is often negative –10

____   In new situations, you're typically not very open-minded –5

____   You don't feel comfortable turning negative situations into positive ones –5

____   You usually let your emotions lead your decision-making –5

____   You're not very open to change and growth opportunities –5

____   Prioritizing tasks and staying focused to completion isn't something you're good at –10

____   You are likely to compare yourself to others - 5

____   Staying on track is hard; you often can't resist temptation or distractions –5

____   You tend to lose motivation when there is a distraction –5

____   A procrastinator, you are unable to manage your time well –5

____   You need other people need to hold you accountable –10

____   You are impulsive and unwilling to delay gratification to achieve goals your –5

____   Stress makes you compromise your self-discipline –10

____   You are susceptible to a fear of failure –10

____   You've had health challenges in the last 6 months that stopped you from doing something you wanted to do –5

____   You're prone to all-or-nothing thinking –5

___ Experiencing failure causes you to lose motivation −5

___ You have trouble adapting to unexpected changes without giving up on your goals −5

___ You view negative experiences as an obstacle rather than opportunities for growth −10

___ You have more examples of giving up than having perseverance −10

___ You give up on your goals too quickly, before giving your efforts a good chance −10

___ You frequently succumb to self-doubt −5

___ Your efforts are inconsistent; sometimes you don't try hard at all −5

___ You lack a deep well of self-love −10

___ You have been unwilling to invest in self-care −10

POINTS TOTAL FOR ALL CHECKED / YES STATEMENTS _____

Tally your final score

Total M+S+R+P (270) − Question total above (80) = sum/4 (47.5)

Percentage + Mentor score (70)/2 = %

Example: 270 − 80 = 190/4 = 47.5

47.5 + 70/2 = **82.5** *(Final score)*

Compare your final score to the percentages below to determine your likelihood to achieve health and wellness goals for life!

86% and above = You have a super high probability of crushing health and weight loss goals. You will make massive, permanent changes to your life and will be able to motivate others to do the same.

83% - 85% = You are a high performer, need very little motivation, are on track to achieve good health and fitness, and don't require accountability.

76% - 82% = You are operating on the high end of crushing goals, you are a true leader, potentially looking for approval, may need some accountability

70% - 75% = You do just enough to get by, need motivation, lack accountability, need approval, will likely not meet long-term goals.

69% and below = You have a mediocre approach to new ideas, not a self-starter, need lots of motivation, lack self-love, and your health and fitness goals are running at a deficit.

Morning five

1. Prayer/devotion: Minimum 10 minutes

2. Exercise/stretch: For at least 10 minutes 3x/week; optimally, stretch, walk or do yoga the other 4 days as well

3. Declarations: These will be based on the opportunities revealed by your MSRP evaluation. Make a list of at least 3 things to declare daily toward healing your life

4. To Do List: This list should include everything that you need to accomplish for the day. Be sure to prioritize the list

5. Detoxification/anti-inflammatory regime: Each morning be sure to complete at least one activity to either detox or anti-inflame your body. Ex: lemon water, water etc.

Night Cap 3

1. Accountability for the morning five

2. Decompress, mind dump

3. Prioritize sleep: Consider going to bed 30 minutes earlier to ensure 7-8 hours of sleep, take whatever steps to ensure that you sleep through the night

   a. Shut technology down ... phones, iPad, TV, etc.

   b. Sleep in a cool, dark room

   c. Maintain consistent sleep schedule

   d. Ensure that you don't eat within 2 hours of going to bed

   e. Consider an Epsom salt bath

Sample 12-minute Exercise: HITT Workouts

Example A

Warm up: 4 twists, 4 squats, 4-second walk in place (repeating the cycle) for a total of 2 minutes.

Do each of the following three exercises for fifty seconds each, with a ten-second rest between each exercise.

1. Squats: hold for 5 seconds, pulse for 5 counts.

2. Hip raises 5 count hold, then 5 pulses

3. High knees

Repeat for 4 rounds.

Example B

Warm up: Jog in place for a total of 2 minutes.

Do each exercise for 50 seconds, rest for 10 seconds, then start the next exercise.

1. In a squat position: 5 1. In a squat position: 5 count arm press, 5 count hold in the middle.

2. Switch jumps.

3. Biceps: 5 count pulsing biceps, 5 count hold in the middle (in the squat position).

Repeat for 4 rounds.

Goal Setting

List 5 goals for each category below that you want to achieve in your life. Then state the timeframe in which you plan to achieve it (in weeks, months, or years)

Spiritual, Health, Personal Growth, Finances, Relationships, Travel

SPIRITUAL/Timeframe	HEALTH/Timeframe
1.	1.
2.	2.
3.	3.
4.	4.
5.	5.
6.	6.

PERSONAL GROWTH/Timeframe	FINANCES/Timeframe
1.	1.
2.	2.
3.	3.
4.	4.
5.	5.
6.	6.

RELATIONSHIPS/Timeframe	TRAVEL/Timeframe
1.	1.
2.	2.
3.	3.
4.	4.
5.	5.
6.	6.

BUILD YOUR TEAM

Think of people who will help support you emotionally, encourage and motivate you, provide practical assistance, give sound advice, hold you accountable, and be instrumental in helping with stress reduction.

1. Family:

2. Friends:

3. Spiritual leader:

4. Functional nutritionist:

5. Mentors/coaches:

6. Therapists/counselors:

7. Primary care physician:

Positive people I spend the most time with:

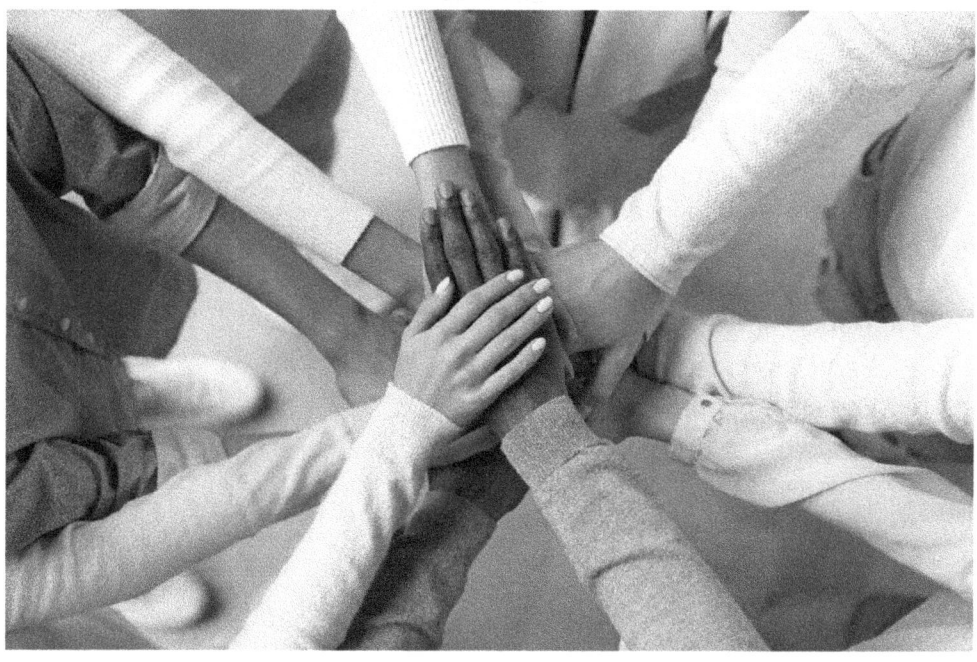

Self-Reflection

Reflecting on these questions can help you assess your level of self-love and identify areas where you may need to cultivate more self-compassion and care. Remember, self-love is a journey, and it takes time and practice to develop a healthy and positive relationship with yourself.

- Do I prioritize my own well-being and happiness?
- Am I kind and compassionate towards myself, especially during challenging times?
- Do I set healthy boundaries and say no when necessary?
- Do I take care of my physical, emotional, and mental health?
- Am I able to forgive myself for past mistakes and learn from them?
- Do I celebrate my achievements and acknowledge my strengths?
- Do I practice self-care and engage in activities that bring me joy and fulfillment?
- Am I able to accept and embrace my flaws and imperfections?
- Do I surround myself with people who uplift and support me?
- Do I believe that I am deserving of love, respect, and happiness?

Here are some ways that we do not love ourselves:

- You criticize yourself
- You conclude that you are unlovable
- You mistreat your body
- You attract people who mistreat you
- You are slow to invest in yourself
- You lack a sense of self-worth
- Often compare yourself to others
- You set unrealistic expectations of yourself
- Participate in negative self-talk
- You are a people pleaser
- Hold on to past mistakes
- Your life is full of chaos and disorder
- You create illness in your body
- You don't believe in yourself

Areas of Opportunity

Opportunity for improvement	How will I get there?	Who's my support team?

Take your health to the next level and prevent or reverse chronic disease!! Scan the QR code below to schedule your free "Strategy Session" to work with Better Choice Health! *Disregard if you have already had your Comprehensive health audit.*

Section 2

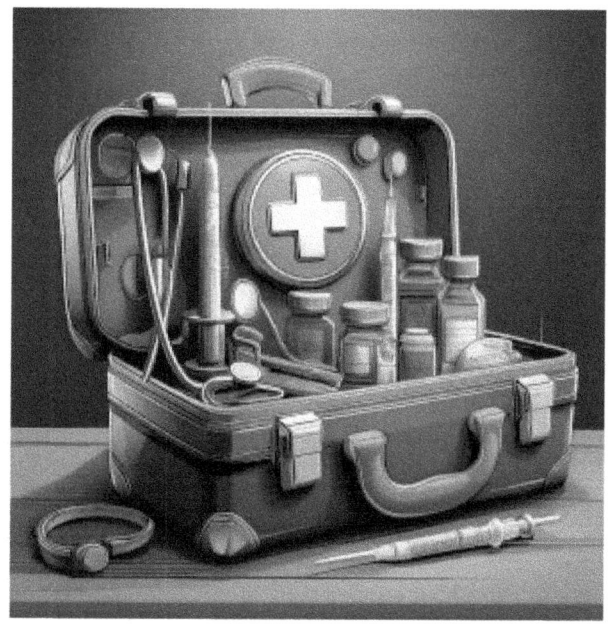

Health Toolkit

Health Toolkit

Blood Glucose Log

Blood Pressure Log

Exercise Tracker

Lab Chart

Symptom Tracker

Weight Tracker

My Records

Family Medical History

My Medical history

Things I am Monitoring

My Physicians

My Advance Directives

Test Results

Action Plan

Blood Glucose Log

Date:	Breakfast Before	Breakfast After	Notes:

Date:	Lunch Before	Lunch After	Notes:

Date:	Dinner Before	Dinner After	Notes:

Normal Blood Sugar Levels

Children to Adolescents; Adults; Elderly

Normal Fasting Glucose (w/out Diabetes)	Fasting Glucose (Consistent with Diabetes)	Target Glucose before meals (w/Type 2 diabetes)	HbA1C (w/out Diabetes)	HbA1C (potential pre-diabetes)	HbA1C with Diabetes	HbA1C (Target goal with diabetes)
Less than or equal to 100mg/dL	Greater than or equal to 126mg/dL	80 to 130 mg/dL	Less than 5.7	5.7 – 6.4	Greater than or equal to 6.5	Less than or equal to 7.0

Fasting vs. Non-Fasting Blood Sugar Levels

Fasting and non-fasting blood sugar tests are used to screen individuals for diabetes and prediabetes.

Fasting blood sugar tests measure blood sugar levels after not having eaten for eight hours and are typically performed in the morning prior to breakfast. Fasting blood sugar levels may indicate that an individual is prediabetic or diabetic based on the following ranges.

- Normal: 99 mg/dL or lower

- Prediabetes: 100 mg/dL to 125 mg/dL

- Diabetes: 126 mg/dL or higher

Non-fasting blood sugar tests don't require an individual to abstain from eating beforehand. Non-fasting blood sugar levels may indicate that an individual is prediabetic or diabetic based on the following ranges.

- Normal: 140 mg/dL or lower

- Prediabetes: 140 mg/dL to 199 mg/dL

- Diabetes: 200 mg/dL or higher

Blood Sugar Levels cont.

Times when you should check your blood sugar:

1. If you are feeling Dizziness

2. If you are sweating excessively

3. If you are experiencing Confusion

4. When you are feeling sick (unexplained)

5. After consuming alcohol

6. Before and after exercise

7. After starting a new medication

8. After taking diabetes medication

Symptoms of high blood sugar levels:

1. Increased thirst

2. Frequent infections

3. Frequent urination

4. Weight loss

5. Listlessness

6. Fatigue

7. Blurred vision

Symptoms of low blood sugar levels:

1. Confusion

2. Dizziness

3. Difficulty concentrating

4. Headache

5. Shaking

6. Sweating

7. Increased heart rate

8. Increased hunger

Dangerous levels for Blood Sugar

Hypoglycemia, Low Blood Sugar

Below 70mg/dL, Severe

Hypoglycemia

Below 54mg/dL

Hyperglycemia, High Blood Sugar

240mg/dL or higher

Blood Sugar Levels, Cont.

When your blood sugar is too low, choose one:

1. Drink 4 ounces of apple or orange juice

2. Drink 4 ounces of soda

3. Take four glucose tablets

4. Eat a few pieces of hard candy

Be sure to test your blood sugar again 15 minutes after implementing one of the suggested methods to raise your blood sugar. If it is still too low, continue trying one of the above treatments.

When your blood sugar is too high: Test your ketone levels, if ketones are normal, you may try one of the below methods to lower your blood sugar levels

1. Get hydrated

2. Engage in physical activity

3. Make sure you are getting enough sleep

4. Manage carbohydrate intake

5. Manage stress levels

Be sure to test your blood sugar again 15 minutes after implementing one of the above methods to lower your blood sugar. If it is still too high, continue trying one of the above treatments and continue to monitor. ***Never hesitate to call your doctor if these methods are not working.

BLOOD PRESSURE TRACKING CHART

Date	Time	Sys*	Dia*	HR*	Date	Time	Sys*	Dia*	HR*

NOTES:

*Systolic (Sys), Diastolic (Dia), Heart Rate (HR)

Exercise and Fitness Tracker

Monthly Stats:						
SUN	MON	TUES	WED	THUR	FRI	SAT
Activity:	Activity:	Activity:	Activity:	Activity:	Activity:	Activity:
Activity:	Activity:	Activity:	Activity:	Activity:	Activity:	Activity:
Activity:	Activity:	Activity:	Activity:	Activity:	Activity:	Activity:
Activity:	Activity:	Activity:	Activity:	Activity:	Activity:	Activity:
Activity:	Activity:	Activity:	Activity:	Activity:	Activity:	Activity:

My Goals!!!   **/ MET:**
1.
2.
3.

MOTIVATION!!!

REWARD:

Lab Chart

*Please note that these are <u>**PATHOLOGICAL RANGES**</u> (used to diagnose disease). To discuss Functional Ranges (used to assess risk for disease before disease develops) reach out to Better Choice Health @ Thebetterchoicehealth.com				
Categories	Your Labs	Minimum	Maximum	Is your lab value within range?
Complete Blood Count (CBC)				
WBC		4.0	10.5	
RBC		3.9	5.1	
Hemoglobin		12.0	16.0	
Hematocrit		36.0	48.2	
RDW		10.8	14.8	
Platelets		150.0	400.0	
Neutrophils		40.0	78.0	
Lymphs		15.0	50.0	
Monocytes		0.0	13.0	
EOS		0.0	5.0	
Basos		0.0	5.0	
Neutrophils (Absolute)				
Lymphs (Absolute)				
Monocytes (Absolute)				
EOS (Absolute)				
Basos (Absolute)				

Categories	Your Labs	Minimum	Maximum	Is your lab value within range?
Complete Metabolic Panel (CMP)				
Glucose, Serum		65.0	110.0	
Uric Acid		1.8	7.0	
BUN		8.0	28.0	
Creatinine, Serum		0.5	1.2	
eGFR				
eGFR (African American)				
BUN/Creation Ratio				
Sodium, Serum		135.0	148.0	
Potassium, Serum		3.5	5.5	
Chloride, Serum		99.0	111.0	
Carbon Dioxide, Total		19.0	31.0	

Categories	Your Labs	Minimum	Maximum	Is your lab value within range?
Calcium, Serum		8.7	10.5	
Phosphorous, Serum		2.3	4.8	
Protein, total serum		6.2	8.3	
Albumin, Serum		3.8	5.0	
Globulin, Total		2.0	3.8	
Bilirubin, Total		0.1	1.5	
Alkaline Phosphatase		27.0	142.0	
LDH		89.0	215.0	
AST		1.0	45.0	
ALT		1.0	55.0	
GGT		5.0	52.0	
Iron, Serum		40.0	180.0	

Categories	Your Labs	Minimum	Maximum	Is your lab value within range?
Complete Metabolic Panel (CMP)				
Glucose, Serum		65.0	110.0	
Uric Acid		1.8	7.0	

BUN		8.0	28.0	
Creatinine, Serum		0.5	1.2	
eGFR				
eGFR (African American)				
BUN/Creatinin Ratio				
Sodium, Serum		135.0	148.0	
Potassium, Serum		3.5	5.5	
Chloride, Serum		99.0	111.0	
Carbon Dioxide, Total		19.0	31.0	
Calcium, Serum		8.7	10.5	
Phosphorous, Serum		2.3	4.8	
Protein, total serum		6.2	8.3	
Albumin, Serum		3.8	5.0	

Globulin, Total		2.0	3.8	
Bilirubin, Total		0.1	1.5	
Alkaline Phosphatase		27.0	142.0	
LDH		89.0	215.0	
AST		1.0	45.0	
ALT		1.0	55.0	
GGT		5.0	52.0	
Iron, Serum		40.0	180.0	
Lipid Panel				
Cholesterol, Total		0.0	200.0	
Triglycerides		35.0	160.0	
HDL Cholesterol		40.0	90.0	
LDL Cholesterol		0.0	130.0	
Total Cholesterol/ HDL Ratio		0.0	3.7	

Additional Markers				
Homocysteine				
Hemoglobin A1C		4.8	5.9	

Insulin (fasting)		2.0	19.0	
TIBC		250.0	390.0	
Transferrin				
Ferritin		33.0	236.0	
Magnesium		1.3	2.3	
C-Reactive (CRP)		0	7.9	
Vitamins				
Vitamin D		32.0	100.0	
Vitamin B12		200.0	1100.0	
Folate		5.5	27.0	
Thyroid Markers				
TSH		0.3	5.7	
Thyroxine		4.5	12.5	
T3 Uptake		27.0	37.0	
Free Thyroxine Index				
Total Triiodothyronnine (TT3)				
Free T3				
Free T4				
Reverse T3				
Thyroid Binding Globulin				
Antithyroglobulin Antibody (TgAb)		0.0	1.0	
Thyroid Perioxidase (TPO) Ab		0.0	34.0	

Symptom Tracker

Symptom	When it Started	Intervention Date	When it ended

Weight Tracker

Start Date/ Goal		Measurement (at the beginning of this journey)	Loss/Gain	End Date/Result
	Weight			
	Left Arm			
	Right Arm			
	Chest			
	Waist			
	Hips			
	Left Thigh			
	Right Thigh			
	Right Thigh			

My Records

Family Medical History

Mother's Side

Name	Relation	Illnesses	*Age/Cause of Death

Father's Side

Name	Relation	Illnesses	*Age/Cause of Death

Immediate Family

Name	Relation	Illnesses	*Age/Cause of Death

*Age at Diagnosis

My Medical History

Condition	Date of diagnosis	Treatment

Past Surgeries:

_____

_____

Things I'm Monitoring

Warning signs	What I need to do

Medical Tracker

Medication: Dosage: Notes:		Medication: Dosage: Notes:		Medication: Dosage: Notes:	
Date:	Time:	Date:	Time:	Date:	Time:

My Physicians

Primary Care Physician:	Phone:
Specialist:	Phone:
Specialist:	Phone:
Specialist:	Phone:
Specialist:	Phone:

Other Contacts

Pharmacy:	Phone:
My Preferred Hospital:	Phone:
Home Health Agency:	Phone:
Others:	Phone:
Transportation:	Phone:

My Advance Directives

___ Yes, I have an Advance Directive

___ No, I do not have an Advance Directive

If yes, where is it located?

_____

Power of Attorney:

_____

Emergency Contact:

Phone:

_____

Relationship:

_____

Test Results

Test/Procedure	Date	Result	Notes	Follow-up

Action Plan

Date:

Nutrition

_____
_____
_____

Supplements

_____
_____
_____

Herbs/Minerals/Superfoods

_____
_____
_____

Lifestyle

_____
_____
_____

Notes:

_____
_____

Section 3

Calendar

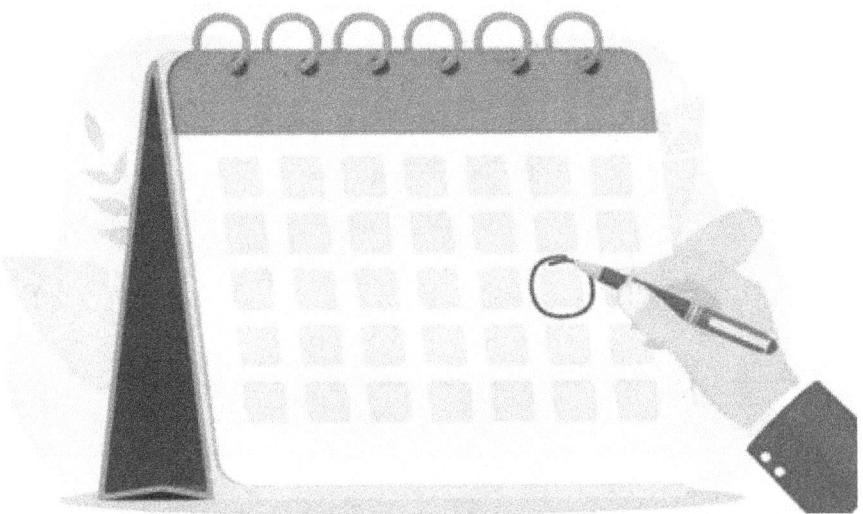

Unlocking Your Health Potential for Life

Month:

Health Goal of the Month:

_____

SUNDAY	MONDAY	TUESDAY	WEDNESDAY	THURSDAY	FRIDAY	SATURDAY

HEALTH TRACKER CHECKLIST

- Physical Activity
- Sleep Tracker
- HR Monitoring
- Blood Pressure
- Blood Sugar
- Nutrition Tracker
- Weight and Body Composition
- Stress and Mood Tracker

ACTION STEPS TO A HEALTHIER YOU:

ACCOUNTABILITY TEAM:

Goal of the Week

To-Do List:

Date _____
Month _____

☐	SUNDAY
☐	MONDAY
☐	TUESDAY
☐	WEDNESDAY
☐	THURSDAY
☐	FRIDAY
☐	SATURDAY

CREATE YOUR ENVIRONMENT/SET UP THE ATMOSPHERE:

WEEKLY REFLECTION:

Morning Five ○○○○○○○
HIIT Workout ○○○
20 Minute Walk ○○○○
Night Cap Three ○○○○○○
Water Goal Met ○○○○○○○

Goal of the Week

To Do List:

Date _____
Month _____

☐ SUNDAY	
☐ MONDAY	
☐ TUESDAY	
☐ WEDNESDAY	
☐ THURSDAY	
☐ FRIDAY	
☐ SATURDAY	

CREATE YOUR ENVIRONMENT/SET UP THE ATMOSPHERE:

_____
_____
_____

WEEKLY REFLECTION:

Morning Five   ○○○○○○○
HIIT Workout   ○○○
20 Minute Walk ○○○○
Night Cap Three ○○○○○○
Water Goal Met   ○○○○○○

Goal of the Week

Date _____
Month _____

To Do List:

☐	SUNDAY	
☐	MONDAY	
☐	TUESDAY	
☐	WEDNESDAY	
☐	THURSDAY	
☐	FRIDAY	
☐	SATURDAY	

WEEKLY REFLECTION:

- Morning Five ○○○○○○○
- HIIT Workout ○○○
- 20 Minute Walk ○○○○
- Night Cap Three ○○○○○○
- Water Goal Met ○○○○○○

CREATE YOUR ENVIRONMENT/SET UP THE ATMOSPHERE:

Goal of the Week

To Do List:

Date _____
Month _____

☐ SUNDAY	
☐ MONDAY	
☐ TUESDAY	
☐ WEDNESDAY	
☐ THURSDAY	
☐ FRIDAY	
☐ SATURDAY	

CREATE YOUR ENVIRONMENT/SET UP THE ATMOSPHERE:

_____
_____
_____
_____

WEEKLY REFLECTION:

_____
_____
_____
_____
_____

Morning Five ○○○○○○○
HIIT Workout ○○○
20 Minute Walk ○○○○
Night Cap Three ○○○○○○
Water Goal Met ○○○○○○

Goal of the Week

To Do List:

Date _____
Month _____

☐	**SUNDAY**
☐	**MONDAY**
☐	**TUESDAY**
☐	**WEDNESDAY**
☐	**THURSDAY**
☐	**FRIDAY**
☐	**SATURDAY**

CREATE YOUR ENVIRONMENT/SET UP THE ATMOSPHERE:

WEEKLY REFLECTION:

- Morning Five ○○○○○○
- HIIT Workout ○○○
- 20 Minute Walk ○○○○
- Night Cap Three ○○○○○○
- Water Goal Met ○○○○○○

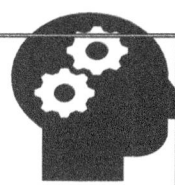

Reflection of the Month

Top 5 victories

1.
2.
3.
4.
5.

What did you learn?

1.
2.
3.
4.

List any setbacks/Obstacles

1.
2.
3.
4.
5.

What health Goals did you accomplish?

1.
2.
3.
4.
5.

What personal goals did you accomplish?

1.
2.
3.
4.
5.

What obstacles did I overcome?

1.
2.
3.
4.

What will I do differently next Month?

1.
2.
3.
4.
5

Month

Health Goal of the Month:

_____

SUNDAY	MONDAY	TUESDAY	WEDNESDAY	THURSDAY	FRIDAY	SATURDAY

HEALTH TRACKER CHECKLIST

- Physical Activity
- Sleep Tracker
- HR Monitoring
- Blood Pressure
- Blood Sugar
- Nutrition Tracker
- Weight and Body Composition
- Stress and Mood Tracker

ACTION STEPS TO A HEALTHIER YOU:

ACCOUNTABILITY TEAM:

Goal of the Week

To Do List:

Date _____
Month _____

☐ SUNDAY	☐ MONDAY	☐ TUESDAY	☐ WEDNESDAY	☐ THURSDAY	☐ FRIDAY	☐ SATURDAY

_____
_____
_____
_____
_____

WEEKLY REFLECTION:

Morning Five ○○○○○○○
HIITT Workout ○○○
20 Minute Walk ○○○○
Night Cap Three ○○○○○○
Water Goal Met ○○○○○○

CREATE YOUR ENVIRONMENT/SET UP THE ATMOSPHERE:

_____
_____
_____
_____

Goal of the Week

To Do List:

Date _____
Month _____

SUNDAY	MONDAY	TUESDAY	WEDNESDAY	THURSDAY	FRIDAY	SATURDAY

CREATE YOUR ENVIRONMENT/SET UP THE ATMOSPHERE:

WEEKLY REFLECTION:

Morning Five ○○○○○○
HIIT Workout ○○○
20 Minute Walk ○○○○
Night Cap Three ○○○○○○
Water Goal Met ○○○○○○

Goal of the Week

To Do List:

Date _____
Month _____

SUNDAY ☐	MONDAY ☐	TUESDAY ☐	WEDNESDAY ☐	THURSDAY ☐	FRIDAY ☐	SATURDAY ☐

WEEKLY REFLECTION:

- Morning Five ○○○○○○○
- HIITT Workout ○○○
- 20 Minute Walk ○○○○
- Night Cap Three ○○○○○○
- Water Goal Met ○○○○○○○

CREATE YOUR ENVIRONMENT/SET UP THE ATMOSPHERE:

Goal of the Week

To Do List:

Date _____
Month _____

☐	SUNDAY
☐	MONDAY
☐	TUESDAY
☐	WEDNESDAY
☐	THURSDAY
☐	FRIDAY
☐	SATURDAY

CREATE YOUR ENVIRONMENT/SET UP THE ATMOSPHERE:

WEEKLY REFLECTION:

- Morning Five ○○○○○○○
- HIIT Workout ○○○
- 20 Minute Walk ○○○○
- Night Cap Three ○○○○○○
- Water Goal Met ○○○○○○

Goal of the Week

To Do List:

Date _____
Month _____

☐	SUNDAY
☐	MONDAY
☐	TUESDAY
☐	WEDNESDAY
☐	THURSDAY
☐	FRIDAY
☐	SATURDAY

CREATE YOUR ENVIRONMENT/SET UP THE ATMOSPHERE:

_____
_____
_____
_____

WEEKLY REFLECTION:

Morning Five ○○○○○○○
HIIT Workout ○○○
20 Minute Walk ○○○
Night Cap Three ○○○○○○
Water Goal Met ○○○○○○○

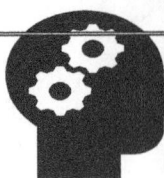

Reflection of the Month

Top 5 victories

1.
2.
3.
4.
5.

What did you learn?

1.
2.
3.
4.

List any setbacks/Obstacles

1.
2.
3.
4.
5.

What health Goals did you accomplish?

1.
2.
3.
4.
5.

What personal goals did you accomplish?

1.
2.
3.
4.
5.

What obstacles did I overcome?

1.
2.
3.
4.

What will I do differently next Month?

1.
2.
3.
4.
5

Month: _____

Health Goal of the Month: _____

SUNDAY	MONDAY	TUESDAY	WEDNESDAY	THURSDAY	FRIDAY	SATURDAY

HEALTH TRACKER CHECKLIST

- Physical Activity
- Sleep Tracker
- HR Monitoring
- Blood Pressure
- Blood Sugar
- Nutrition Tracker
- Weight and Body Composition
- Stress and Mood Tracker

ACTION STEPS TO A HEALTHIER YOU:

_____
_____
_____
_____
_____

ACCOUNTABILITY TEAM:

_____
_____

Goal of the Week

To Do List:

Date _____
Month _____

☐	SUNDAY
☐	MONDAY
☐	TUESDAY
☐	WEDNESDAY
☐	THURSDAY
☐	FRIDAY
☐	SATURDAY

CREATE YOUR ENVIRONMENT/SET UP THE ATMOSPHERE:

WEEKLY REFLECTION:

Morning Five ○○○○○○○
HIIT Workout ○○○
20 Minute Walk ○○○○
Night Cap Three ○○○○○○
Water Goal Met ○○○○○○

Goal of the Week

To Do List:

Date _____
Month _____

☐	SUNDAY
☐	MONDAY
☐	TUESDAY
☐	WEDNESDAY
☐	THURSDAY
☐	FRIDAY
☐	SATURDAY

CREATE YOUR ENVIRONMENT/SET UP THE ATMOSPHERE:

_____
_____
_____
_____

WEEKLY REFLECTION:

Morning Five ○○○○○○
HIIT Workout ○○○
20 Minute Walk ○○○○
Night Cap Three ○○○○○○
Water Goal Met ○○○○○○

Goal of the Week

To Do List:

Date _____
Month _____

SUNDAY ☐	MONDAY ☐	TUESDAY ☐	WEDNESDAY ☐	THURSDAY ☐	FRIDAY ☐	SATURDAY ☐

CREATE YOUR ENVIRONMENT/SET UP THE ATMOSPHERE:

_____
_____
_____
_____

WEEKLY REFLECTION:

- Morning Five ○○○○○○○
- HIIT Workout ○○○
- 20 Minute Walk ○○○○
- Night Cap Three ○○○○○○○
- Water Goal Met ○○○○○○○

Goal of the Week

To Do List:

Date _____
Month _____

SUNDAY ☐	
MONDAY ☐	
TUESDAY ☐	
WEDNESDAY ☐	
THURSDAY ☐	
FRIDAY ☐	
SATURDAY ☐	

CREATE YOUR ENVIRONMENT/SET UP THE ATMOSPHERE:

WEEKLY REFLECTION:

Morning Five ○○○○○○○
HIIT Workout ○○○
20 Minute Walk ○○○
Night Cap Three ○○○○○○
Water Goal Met ○○○○○○○

Goal of the Week

To Do List:

Date _____
Month _____

☐ SUNDAY	
☐ MONDAY	
☐ TUESDAY	
☐ WEDNESDAY	
☐ THURSDAY	
☐ FRIDAY	
☐ SATURDAY	

CREATE YOUR ENVIRONMENT/SET UP THE ATMOSPHERE:

_____
_____
_____
_____
_____

WEEKLY REFLECTION:

Morning Five ○○○○○○○
HIIT Workout ○○○
20 Minute Walk ○○○○
Night Cap Three ○○○○○○
Water Goal Met ○○○○○○○

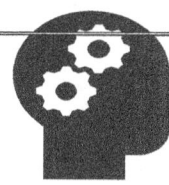

Reflection of the Month

Top 5 victories

1.
2.
3.
4.
5.

What did you learn?

1.
2.
3.
4.

List any setbacks/Obstacles

1.
2.
3.
4.
5.

What health Goals did you accomplish?

1.
2.
3.
4.
5.

What personal goals did you accomplish?

1.
2.
3.
4.
5.

What obstacles did I overcome?

1.
2.
3.
4.

What will I do differently next Month?

1.
2.
3.
4.
5

Month: _____

Health Goal of the Month: _____

	SUNDAY	MONDAY	TUESDAY	WEDNESDAY	THURSDAY	FRIDAY	SATURDAY

HEALTH TRACKER CHECKLIST

- Physical Activity
- Sleep Tracker
- HR Monitoring
- Blood Pressure
- Blood Sugar
- Nutrition Tracker
- Weight and Body Composition
- Stress and Mood Tracker

ACTION STEPS TO A HEALTHIER YOU:

_____
_____
_____

ACCOUNTABILITY TEAM:

_____
_____
_____

Goal of the Week

Date _____
Month _____

To Do list:

SUNDAY ☐	MONDAY ☐	TUESDAY ☐	WEDNESDAY ☐	THURSDAY ☐	FRIDAY ☐	SATURDAY ☐

CREATE YOUR ENVIRONMENT/SET UP THE ATMOSPHERE:

_____
_____
_____
_____

WEEKLY REFLECTION:

- Morning Five ○○○○○○
- HIIT Workout ○○○
- 20 Minute Walk ○○○
- Night Cap Three ○○○○○○
- Water Goal Met ○○○○○○

Goal of the Week

To Do List:

Date _____
Month _____

☐	SUNDAY
☐	MONDAY
☐	TUESDAY
☐	WEDNESDAY
☐	THURSDAY
☐	FRIDAY
☐	SATURDAY

CREATE YOUR ENVIRONMENT/SET UP THE ATMOSPHERE:

WEEKLY REFLECTION:

Morning Five ○○○○○○○
HIIT Workout ○○○
20 Minute Walk ○○○○
Night Cap Three ○○○○○○
Water Goal Met ○○○○○○○

Goal of the Week

To Do List:

Date _____
Month _____

SUNDAY ☐	MONDAY ☐	TUESDAY ☐	WEDNESDAY ☐	THURSDAY ☐	FRIDAY ☐	SATURDAY ☐

CREATE YOUR ENVIRONMENT/SET UP THE ATMOSPHERE:

_____
_____
_____

WEEKLY REFLECTION:

_____
_____
_____

- **Morning Five** ○○○○○○○
- **HIIT Workout** ○○○
- **20 Minute Walk** ○○○○
- **Night Cap Three** ○○○○○○
- **Water Goal Met** ○○○○○○○

Goal of the Week

Date _____
Month _____

To Do List:
_____
_____
_____
_____
_____
_____
_____

☐ SUNDAY	
☐ MONDAY	
☐ TUESDAY	
☐ WEDNESDAY	
☐ THURSDAY	
☐ FRIDAY	
☐ SATURDAY	

CREATE YOUR ENVIRONMENT/SET UP THE ATMOSPHERE:
_____
_____

WEEKLY REFLECTION:
_____
_____
_____
_____

- Morning Five ○○○○○○
- HIIT Workout ○○○
- 20 Minute Walk ○○○○
- Night Cap Three ○○○○○○
- Water Goal Met ○○○○○○

Goal of the Week

Date _____
Month _____

To Do List:
- _____
- _____
- _____
- _____
- _____
- _____

☐ SUNDAY	☐ MONDAY	☐ TUESDAY	☐ WEDNESDAY	☐ THURSDAY	☐ FRIDAY	☐ SATURDAY

CREATE YOUR ENVIRONMENT/SET UP THE ATMOSPHERE:
_____
_____
_____

WEEKLY REFLECTION:

Morning Five ○○○○○○○
HIIT Workout ○○○
20 Minute Walk ○○○○
Night Cap Three ○○○○○○
Water Goal Met ○○○○○○○

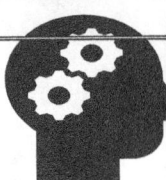

Reflection of the Month

Top 5 victories

1.
2.
3.
4.
5.

What did you learn?

1.
2.
3.
4.

List any setbacks/Obstacles

1.
2.
3.
4.
5.

What health Goals did you accomplish?

1.
2.
3.
4.
5.

What personal goals did you accomplish?

1.
2.
3.
4.
5.

What obstacles did I overcome?

1.
2.
3.
4.

What will I do differently next Month?

1.
2.
3.
4.
5

Reflection of the Month

Month:

Health Goal of the Month: _____

SUNDAY	MONDAY	TUESDAY	WEDNESDAY	THURSDAY	FRIDAY	SATURDAY

HEALTH TRACKER CHECKLIST
- Physical Activity
- Sleep Tracker
- HR Monitoring
- Blood Pressure
- Blood Sugar
- Nutrition Tracker
- Weight and Body Composition
- Stress and Mood Tracker

ACTION STEPS TO A HEALTHIER YOU:

ACCOUNTABILITY TEAM:

Goal of the Week

To Do List:

Date _____
Month _____

SUNDAY	MONDAY	TUESDAY	WEDNESDAY	THURSDAY	FRIDAY	SATURDAY
☐	☐	☐	☐	☐	☐	☐

WEEKLY REFLECTION:

Morning Five ◯◯◯◯◯◯◯
HIIT Workout ◯◯◯
20 Minute Walk ◯◯◯◯
Night Cap Three ◯◯◯◯◯◯
Water Goal Met ◯◯◯◯◯◯◯

CREATE YOUR ENVIRONMENT/SET UP THE ATMOSPHERE:

Goal of the Week

To Do List:

Date _____
Month _____

☐ SUNDAY	
☐ MONDAY	
☐ TUESDAY	
☐ WEDNESDAY	
☐ THURSDAY	
☐ FRIDAY	
☐ SATURDAY	

CREATE YOUR ENVIRONMENT/SET UP THE ATMOSPHERE:

_____
_____
_____

WEEKLY REFLECTION:

Morning Five ○○○○○○○
HIIT Workout ○○○
20 Minute Walk ○○○○
Night Cap Three ○○○○○○
Water Goal Met ○○○○○○○

Goal of the Week

To Do List:

Date _____
Month _____

	SUNDAY	MONDAY	TUESDAY	WEDNESDAY	THURSDAY	FRIDAY	SATURDAY
☐							

CREATE YOUR ENVIRONMENT/SET UP THE ATMOSPHERE:

_____
_____
_____
_____

WEEKLY REFLECTION:

Morning Five   ○○○○○○○
HIIT Workout   ○○○
20 Minute Walk ○○○○
Night Cap Three ○○○○○○
Water Goal Met ○○○○○○○

_____
_____
_____
_____

Goal of the Week

To Do List:

Date _____
Month _____

☐ SUNDAY	
☐ MONDAY	
☐ TUESDAY	
☐ WEDNESDAY	
☐ THURSDAY	
☐ FRIDAY	
☐ SATURDAY	

CREATE YOUR ENVIRONMENT/SET UP THE ATMOSPHERE:

_____
_____
_____
_____

WEEKLY REFLECTION:

- Morning Five ○○○○○○○
- HIIT Workout ○○○
- 20 Minute Walk ○○○○
- Night Cap Three ○○○○○○
- Water Goal Met ○○○○○○○

Goal of the Week

To Do List:

_____
_____
_____
_____
_____
_____
_____

Date _____
Month _____

☐ SUNDAY	
☐ MONDAY	
☐ TUESDAY	
☐ WEDNESDAY	
☐ THURSDAY	
☐ FRIDAY	
☐ SATURDAY	

CREATE YOUR ENVIRONMENT/SET UP THE ATMOSPHERE:

WEEKLY REFLECTION:

Morning Five ○○○○○○○
HIIT Workout ○○○
20 Minute Walk ○○○○
Night Cap Three ○○○○○○
Water Goal Met ○○○○○○

_____
_____
_____
_____
_____
_____

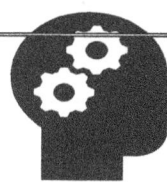

Top 5 victories

1.
2.
3.
4.
5.

What did you learn?

1.
2.
3.
4.

List any setbacks/Obstacles

1.
2.
3.
4.
5.

What health Goals did you accomplish?

1.
2.
3.
4.
5.

What personal goals did you accomplish?

1.
2.
3.
4.
5.

What obstacles did I overcome?

1.
2.
3.
4.

What will I do differently next Month?

1.
2.
3.
4.
5

Month: _____

Health Goal of the Month: _____

___	___	___	___	___

HEALTH TRACKER CHECKLIST

- Physical Activity
- Sleep Tracker
- HR Monitoring
- Blood Pressure
- Blood Sugar
- Nutrition Tracker
- Weight and Body Composition
- Stress and Mood Tracker

SUNDAY	MONDAY	TUESDAY	WEDNESDAY	THURSDAY	FRIDAY	SATURDAY

ACTION STEPS TO A HEALTHIER YOU:

ACCOUNTABILITY TEAM:

Goal of the Week

To Do List:

Date _____
Month _____

☐	SUNDAY
☐	MONDAY
☐	TUESDAY
☐	WEDNESDAY
☐	THURSDAY
☐	FRIDAY
☐	SATURDAY

CREATE YOUR ENVIRONMENT/SET UP THE ATMOSPHERE:

_____
_____
_____
_____
_____

WEEKLY REFLECTION:

Morning Five ○○○○○○○
HIITT Workout ○○○
20 Minute Walk ○○○
Night Cap Three ○○○○○○
Water Goal Met ○○○○○○

Goal of the Week

To Do List:

Date _____
Month _____

SUNDAY ☐	MONDAY ☐	TUESDAY ☐	WEDNESDAY ☐	THURSDAY ☐	FRIDAY ☐	SATURDAY ☐

CREATE YOUR ENVIRONMENT/SET UP THE ATMOSPHERE:

_____
_____
_____
_____

WEEKLY REFLECTION:

- Morning Five ○○○○○○
- HIIT Workout ○○○
- 20 Minute Walk ○○○○
- Night Cap Three ○○○○○○
- Water Goal Met ○○○○○○

_____
_____
_____
_____

Goal of the Week

To Do List:

Date _____
Month _____

SUNDAY ☐	MONDAY ☐	TUESDAY ☐	WEDNESDAY ☐	THURSDAY ☐	FRIDAY ☐	SATURDAY ☐

_____
_____
_____
_____
_____
_____

CREATE YOUR ENVIRONMENT/SET UP THE ATMOSPHERE:

_____
_____

WEEKLY REFLECTION:

Morning Five ○○○○○○○
HIITT Workout ○○○
20 Minute Walk ○○○○
Night Cap Three ○○○○○○○
Water Goal Met ○○○○○○○

Goal of the Week

To Do List:

Date _____
Month _____

☐ SUNDAY		
☐ MONDAY		
☐ TUESDAY		
☐ WEDNESDAY		
☐ THURSDAY		
☐ FRIDAY		
☐ SATURDAY		

CREATE YOUR ENVIRONMENT/SET UP THE ATMOSPHERE:

_____
_____
_____
_____

WEEKLY REFLECTION:

Morning Five   ○○○○○○○
HIIT Workout   ○○○
20 Minute Walk   ○○○○
Night Cap Three ○○○○○○
Water Goal Met   ○○○○○○○

Goal of the Week

Date _____
Month _____

To Do List:

☐ SUNDAY	
☐ MONDAY	
☐ TUESDAY	
☐ WEDNESDAY	
☐ THURSDAY	
☐ FRIDAY	
☐ SATURDAY	

CREATE YOUR ENVIRONMENT/SET UP THE ATMOSPHERE:

_____
_____
_____

WEEKLY REFLECTION:

Morning Five ○○○○○○○
HIIT Workout ○○○
20 Minute Walk ○○○
Night Cap Three ○○○○○○
Water Goal Met ○○○○○○

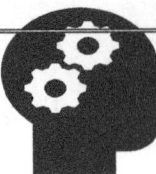

Reflection of the Month

Top 5 victories

1.
2.
3.
4.
5.

What did you learn?

1.
2.
3.
4.

List any setbacks/Obstacles

1.
2.
3.
4.
5.

What health Goals did you accomplish?

1.
2.
3.
4.
5.

What personal goals did you accomplish?

1.
2.
3.
4.
5.

What obstacles did I overcome?

1.
2.
3.
4.

What will I do differently next Month?

1.
2.
3.
4.
5

Month:

Health Goal of the Month:

SUNDAY	MONDAY	TUESDAY	WEDNESDAY	THURSDAY	FRIDAY	SATURDAY

ACTION STEPS TO A HEALTHIER YOU:

ACCOUNTABILITY TEAM:

HEALTH TRACKER CHECKLIST

- Physical Activity
- Sleep Tracker
- HR Monitoring
- Blood Pressure
- Blood Sugar
- Nutrition Tracker
- Weight and Body Composition
- Stress and Mood Tracker

Goal of the Week

To Do List:

Date ―――
Month ―――

SUNDAY	MONDAY	TUESDAY	WEDNESDAY	THURSDAY	FRIDAY	SATURDAY
☐	☐	☐	☐	☐	☐	☐

WEEKLY REFLECTION:

- Morning Five ○○○○○○
- HIIT Workout ○○○
- 20 Minute Walk ○○○○
- Night Cap Three ○○○○○
- Water Goal Met ○○○○○

CREATE YOUR ENVIRONMENT/SET UP THE ATMOSPHERE:

Goal of the Week

To Do List:

Date _____
Month _____

☐ SUNDAY	
☐ MONDAY	
☐ TUESDAY	
☐ WEDNESDAY	
☐ THURSDAY	
☐ FRIDAY	
☐ SATURDAY	

CREATE YOUR ENVIRONMENT/SET UP THE ATMOSPHERE:

_____
_____
_____
_____
_____
_____
_____

WEEKLY REFLECTION:

- Morning Five ○○○○○○○
- HIIT Workout ○○○
- 20 Minute Walk ○○○○
- Night Cap Three ○○○○○○
- Water Goal Met ○○○○○○

Goal of the Week

To Do List:

Date _____
Month _____

	SUNDAY	MONDAY	TUESDAY	WEDNESDAY	THURSDAY	FRIDAY	SATURDAY
☐							

CREATE YOUR ENVIRONMENT/SET UP THE ATMOSPHERE:

_____
_____
_____
_____

WEEKLY REFLECTION:

- Morning Five ○○○○○○
- HIIT Workout ○○○
- 20 Minute Walk ○○○○
- Night Cap Three ○○○○○○
- Water Goal Met ○○○○○○

Goal of the Week

To Do List:

Date _____
Month _____

☐	**SUNDAY**
☐	**MONDAY**
☐	**TUESDAY**
☐	**WEDNESDAY**
☐	**THURSDAY**
☐	**FRIDAY**
☐	**SATURDAY**

CREATE YOUR ENVIRONMENT/SET UP THE ATMOSPHERE:

_____
_____
_____
_____

WEEKLY REFLECTION:

- **Morning Five** ○○○○○○○
- **HIIT Workout** ○○○
- **20 Minute Walk** ○○○○
- **Night Cap Three** ○○○○○○
- **Water Goal Met** ○○○○○○

Goal of the Week

Date _____
Month _____

To Do List:

☐ SUNDAY	☐ MONDAY	☐ TUESDAY	☐ WEDNESDAY	☐ THURSDAY	☐ FRIDAY	☐ SATURDAY

CREATE YOUR ENVIRONMENT/SET UP THE ATMOSPHERE:

_____
_____
_____
_____

WEEKLY REFLECTION:

- Morning Five ○○○○○○○
- HIIT Workout ○○○
- 20 Minute Walk ○○○○
- Night Cap Three ○○○○○○
- Water Goal Met ○○○○○○

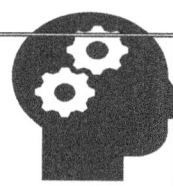

Reflection of the Month

Top 5 victories

1.
2.
3.
4.
5.

What did you learn?

1.
2.
3.
4.

List any setbacks/Obstacles

1.
2.
3.
4.
5.

What health Goals did you accomplish?

1.
2.
3.
4.
5.

What personal goals did you accomplish?

1.
2.
3.
4.
5.

What obstacles did I overcome?

1.
2.
3.
4.

What will I do differently next Month?

1.
2.
3.
4.
5

Month:

Health Goal of the Month:

_____
_____
_____
_____
_____

HEALTH TRACKER CHECKLIST

- Physical Activity
- Sleep Tracker
- HR Monitoring
- Blood Pressure
- Blood Sugar
- Nutrition Tracker
- Weight and Body Composition
- Stress and Mood Tracker

ACTION STEPS TO A HEALTHIER YOU:

ACCOUNTABILITY TEAM:

SUNDAY	MONDAY	TUESDAY	WEDNESDAY	THURSDAY	FRIDAY	SATURDAY

Goal of the Week
To Do List:

Date _____
Month _____

☐	SUNDAY
☐	MONDAY
☐	TUESDAY
☐	WEDNESDAY
☐	THURSDAY
☐	FRIDAY
☐	SATURDAY

WEEKLY REFLECTION:

Morning Five ○○○○○○○
HIIT Workout ○○○
20 Minute Walk ○○○○
Night Cap Three ○○○○○○○
Water Goal Met ○○○○○○○

CREATE YOUR ENVIRONMENT/SET UP THE ATMOSPHERE:

Goal of the Week

Date _____
Month _____

To Do List:

☐	**SUNDAY**
☐	**MONDAY**
☐	**TUESDAY**
☐	**WEDNESDAY**
☐	**THURSDAY**
☐	**FRIDAY**
☐	**SATURDAY**

CREATE YOUR ENVIRONMENT/SET UP THE ATMOSPHERE:

_____
_____
_____
_____
_____
_____

WEEKLY REFLECTION:

- Morning Five ○○○○○○
- HIIT Workout ○○○
- 20 Minute Walk ○○○○
- Night Cap Three ○○○○○○
- Water Goal Met ○○○○○○

Goal of the Week

To Do List:

Date _____
Month _____

☐	SUNDAY
☐	MONDAY
☐	TUESDAY
☐	WEDNESDAY
☐	THURSDAY
☐	FRIDAY
☐	SATURDAY

CREATE YOUR ENVIRONMENT/SET UP THE ATMOSPHERE:

WEEKLY REFLECTION:

- **Morning Five** ○○○○○○○
- **HIIT Workout** ○○○
- **20 Minute Walk** ○○○○
- **Night Cap Three** ○○○○○○○
- **Water Goal Met** ○○○○○○○

Goal of the Week

To Do List:

Date _____
Month _____

□	SUNDAY	
□	MONDAY	
□	TUESDAY	
□	WEDNESDAY	
□	THURSDAY	
□	FRIDAY	
□	SATURDAY	

WEEKLY REFLECTION:

- Morning Five ○○○○○○○
- HIIT Workout ○○○
- 20 Minute Walk ○○○○
- Night Cap Three ○○○○○○○
- Water Goal Met ○○○○○○○

CREATE YOUR ENVIRONMENT/SET UP THE ATMOSPHERE:

Goal of the Week

To Do List:

Date _____
Month _____

☐ SUNDAY	
☐ MONDAY	
☐ TUESDAY	
☐ WEDNESDAY	
☐ THURSDAY	
☐ FRIDAY	
☐ SATURDAY	

CREATE YOUR ENVIRONMENT/SET UP THE ATMOSPHERE:

_____
_____
_____
_____
_____

WEEKLY REFLECTION:

Morning Five ○○○○○○○
HIIT Workout ○○○
20 Minute Walk ○○○
Night Cap Three ○○○○○○○
Water Goal Met ○○○○○○○

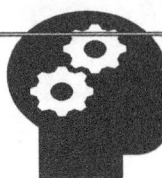

Reflection of the Month

Top 5 victories

1.
2.
3.
4.
5.

What did you learn?

1.
2.
3.
4.

List any setbacks/Obstacles

1.
2.
3.
4.
5.

What health Goals did you accomplish?

1.
2.
3.
4.
5.

What personal goals did you accomplish?

1.
2.
3.
4.
5.

What obstacles did I overcome?

1.
2.
3.
4.

What will I do differently next Month?

1.
2.
3.
4.
5

Month

Health Goal of the Month: _____

SUNDAY	MONDAY	TUESDAY	WEDNESDAY	THURSDAY	FRIDAY	SATURDAY

HEALTH TRACKER CHECKLIST

- Physical Activity
- Sleep Tracker
- HR Monitoring
- Blood Pressure
- Blood Sugar
- Nutrition Tracker
- Weight and Body Composition
- Stress and Mood Tracker

ACTION STEPS TO A HEALTHIER YOU:

_____
_____
_____

ACCOUNTABILITY TEAM:

_____
_____
_____

Goal of the Week

To Do List:

Date _____
Month _____

SUNDAY ☐	
MONDAY ☐	
TUESDAY ☐	
WEDNESDAY ☐	
THURSDAY ☐	
FRIDAY ☐	
SATURDAY ☐	

WEEKLY REFLECTION:

Morning Five ○○○○○○○
HIIT Workout ○○○
20 Minute Walk ○○○○
Night Cap Three ○○○○○○
Water Goal Met ○○○○○○○

CREATE YOUR ENVIRONMENT/SET UP THE ATMOSPHERE:

Goal of the Week

To-Do List:

Date _____
Month _____

☐	SUNDAY
☐	MONDAY
☐	TUESDAY
☐	WEDNESDAY
☐	THURSDAY
☐	FRIDAY
☐	SATURDAY

WEEKLY REFLECTION:

- Morning Five ○○○○○○○
- HIITT Workout ○○○
- 20 Minute Walk ○○○○
- Night Cap Three ○○○○○○○
- Water Goal Met ○○○○○○○

CREATE YOUR ENVIRONMENT/SET UP THE ATMOSPHERE:

Goal of the Week

To Do List:

Date _____
Month _____

☐	SUNDAY
☐	MONDAY
☐	TUESDAY
☐	WEDNESDAY
☐	THURSDAY
☐	FRIDAY
☐	SATURDAY

CREATE YOUR ENVIRONMENT/SET UP THE ATMOSPHERE:

WEEKLY REFLECTION:

- Morning Five ○○○○○○
- HIIT Workout ○○○
- 20 Minute Walk ○○○○
- Night Cap Three ○○○○○○
- Water Goal Met ○○○○○○

Goal of the Week

To Do List:

Date _____
Month _____

☐	**SUNDAY**
☐	**MONDAY**
☐	**TUESDAY**
☐	**WEDNESDAY**
☐	**THURSDAY**
☐	**FRIDAY**
☐	**SATURDAY**

CREATE YOUR ENVIRONMENT/SET UP THE ATMOSPHERE:

WEEKLY REFLECTION:

- **Morning Five** ○○○○○○○
- **HIIT Workout** ○○○
- **20 Minute Walk** ○○○○
- **Night Cap Three** ○○○○○○
- **Water Goal Met** ○○○○○○○

Goal of the Week

To Do List:

Date _____
Month _____

☐	SUNDAY
☐	MONDAY
☐	TUESDAY
☐	WEDNESDAY
☐	THURSDAY
☐	FRIDAY
☐	SATURDAY

CREATE YOUR ENVIRONMENT/SET UP THE ATMOSPHERE:

WEEKLY REFLECTION:

- Morning Five ○○○○○○
- HIIT Workout ○○○
- 20 Minute Walk ○○○○
- Night Cap Three ○○○○○○
- Water Goal Met ○○○○○○

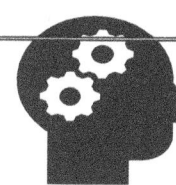

Reflection of the Month

Top 5 victories

1.
2.
3.
4.
5.

What did you learn?

1.
2.
3.
4.

List any setbacks/Obstacles

1.
2.
3.
4.
5.

What health Goals did you accomplish?

1.
2.
3.
4.
5.

What personal goals did you accomplish?

1.
2.
3.
4.
5.

What obstacles did I overcome?

1.
2.
3.
4.

What will I do differently next Month?

1.
2.
3.
4.
5

Month:

Health Goal of the Month:

_____

SUNDAY	MONDAY	TUESDAY	WEDNESDAY	THURSDAY	FRIDAY	SATURDAY

HEALTH TRACKER CHECKLIST

- Physical Activity
- Sleep Tracker
- HR Monitoring
- Blood Pressure
- Blood Sugar
- Nutrition Tracker
- Weight and Body Composition
- Stress and Mood Tracker

ACTION STEPS TO A HEALTHIER YOU:

ACCOUNTABILITY TEAM:

Goal of the Week

To Do List:

Date _____
Month _____

☐ SUNDAY	
☐ MONDAY	
☐ TUESDAY	
☐ WEDNESDAY	
☐ THURSDAY	
☐ FRIDAY	
☐ SATURDAY	

CREATE YOUR ENVIRONMENT/SET UP THE ATMOSPHERE:

_____
_____
_____
_____
_____

WEEKLY REFLECTION:

- Morning Five ○○○○○○○
- HIIT Workout ○○○
- 20 Minute Walk ○○○○
- Night Cap Three ○○○○○○○
- Water Goal Met ○○○○○○○

Goal of the Week

To Do List:

Date _____
Month _____

SUNDAY	MONDAY	TUESDAY	WEDNESDAY	THURSDAY	FRIDAY	SATURDAY

CREATE YOUR ENVIRONMENT/SET UP THE ATMOSPHERE:

WEEKLY REFLECTION:

Morning Five ○○○○○○○
HIIT Workout ○○○
20 Minute Walk ○○○○
Night Cap Three ○○○○○○○
Water Goal Met ○○○○○○○

Goal of the Week

To Do List:

Date _____
Month _____

☐ SUNDAY	
☐ MONDAY	
☐ TUESDAY	
☐ WEDNESDAY	
☐ THURSDAY	
☐ FRIDAY	
☐ SATURDAY	

CREATE YOUR ENVIRONMENT/SET UP THE ATMOSPHERE:

_____
_____
_____
_____

WEEKLY REFLECTION:

Morning Five ○○○○○○○
HIIT Workout ○○○
20 Minute Walk ○○○○
Night Cap Three ○○○○○○
Water Goal Met ○○○○○○

Goal of the Week

To Do List:

Date _____
Month _____

	SUNDAY	MONDAY	TUESDAY	WEDNESDAY	THURSDAY	FRIDAY	SATURDAY
☐							

CREATE YOUR ENVIRONMENT/SET UP THE ATMOSPHERE:

_____
_____
_____
_____
_____
_____

WEEKLY REFLECTION:

Morning Five ○○○○○○○
HIIT Workout ○○○
20 Minute Walk ○○○○
Night Cap Three ○○○○○○
Water Goal Met ○○○○○○

Goal of the Week

To Do List:

Date _____
Month _____

☐ SUNDAY	☐ MONDAY	☐ TUESDAY	☐ WEDNESDAY	☐ THURSDAY	☐ FRIDAY	☐ SATURDAY

WEEKLY REFLECTION:

- Morning Five ○○○○○○○
- HIIT Workout ○○○
- 20 Minute Walk ○○○○
- Night Cap Three ○○○○○○
- Water Goal Met ○○○○○○

CREATE YOUR ENVIRONMENT/SET UP THE ATMOSPHERE:

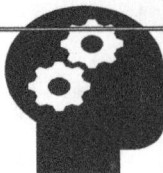

Reflection of the Month

Top 5 victories

1.
2.
3.
4.
5.

What did you learn?

1.
2.
3.
4.

List any setbacks/Obstacles

1.
2.
3.
4.
5.

What health Goals did you accomplish?

1.
2.
3.

4.
5.

What personal goals did you accomplish?

1.
2.
3.
4.
5.

What obstacles did I overcome?

1.
2.
3.
4.

What will I do differently next Month?

1.
2.
3.
4.
5

Month:

Health Goal of the Month:

_____
_____
_____
_____
_____

SUNDAY	MONDAY	TUESDAY	WEDNESDAY	THURSDAY	FRIDAY	SATURDAY

HEALTH TRACKER CHECKLIST

- Physical Activity
- Sleep Tracker
- HR Monitoring
- Blood Pressure
- Blood Sugar
- Nutrition Tracker
- Weight and Body Composition
- Stress and Mood Tracker

ACTION STEPS TO A HEALTHIER YOU:

ACCOUNTABILITY TEAM:

Goal of the Week

To Do List:

Date _____
Month _____

SUNDAY ☐	
MONDAY ☐	
TUESDAY ☐	
WEDNESDAY ☐	
THURSDAY ☐	
FRIDAY ☐	
SATURDAY ☐	

CREATE YOUR ENVIRONMENT/SET UP THE ATMOSPHERE:

_____
_____
_____
_____

WEEKLY REFLECTION:

Morning Five ○○○○○○
HIITT Workout ○○○
20 Minute Walk ○○○○
Night Cap Three ○○○○○○
Water Goal Met ○○○○○○

Goal of the Week

To Do List:

Date _____
Month _____

☐	SUNDAY
☐	MONDAY
☐	TUESDAY
☐	WEDNESDAY
☐	THURSDAY
☐	FRIDAY
☐	SATURDAY

CREATE YOUR ENVIRONMENT/SET UP THE ATMOSPHERE:

WEEKLY REFLECTION:

Morning Five ○○○○○○○
HIIT Workout ○○○
20 Minute Walk ○○○○
Night Cap Three ○○○○○○
Water Goal Met ○○○○○○

Goal of the Week

To Do List:

Date _____
Month _____

☐	SUNDAY	
☐	MONDAY	
☐	TUESDAY	
☐	WEDNESDAY	
☐	THURSDAY	
☐	FRIDAY	
☐	SATURDAY	

CREATE YOUR ENVIRONMENT/SET UP THE ATMOSPHERE:

_____
_____
_____
_____
_____

WEEKLY REFLECTION:

- Morning Five ○○○○○○
- HIIT Workout ○○○
- 20 Minute Walk ○○○○
- Night Cap Three ○○○○○○
- Water Goal Met ○○○○○○

Goal of the Week

To Do List:

Date _____
Month _____

☐ SUNDAY	
☐ MONDAY	
☐ TUESDAY	
☐ WEDNESDAY	
☐ THURSDAY	
☐ FRIDAY	
☐ SATURDAY	

CREATE YOUR ENVIRONMENT/SET UP THE ATMOSPHERE:

WEEKLY REFLECTION:

Morning Five ○○○○○○
HIIT Workout ○○○
20 Minute Walk ○○○○
Night Cap Three ○○○○○○
Water Goal Met ○○○○○○

Goal of the Week

To Do List:

Date _____
Month _____

SUNDAY ☐	MONDAY ☐	TUESDAY ☐	WEDNESDAY ☐	THURSDAY ☐	FRIDAY ☐	SATURDAY ☐

CREATE YOUR ENVIRONMENT/SET UP THE ATMOSPHERE:

_____
_____
_____
_____

WEEKLY REFLECTION:

- Morning Five ○○○○○○○
- HIITT Workout ○○○
- 20 Minute Walk ○○○○
- Night Cap Three ○○○○○○
- Water Goal Met ○○○○○○

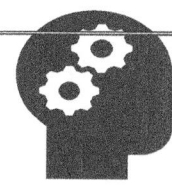

Reflection of the Month

Top 5 victories

1.
2.
3.
4.
5.

What did you learn?

1.
2.
3.
4.

List any setbacks/Obstacles

1.
2.
3.
4.
5.

What health Goals did you accomplish?

1.
2.
3.
4.
5.

What personal goals did you accomplish?

1.
2.
3.
4.
5.

What obstacles did I overcome?

1.
2.
3.
4.

What will I do differently next Month?

1.
2.
3.
4.
5

Month: _____

Health Goal of the Month: _____

	SUNDAY	MONDAY	TUESDAY	WEDNESDAY	THURSDAY	FRIDAY	SATURDAY

HEALTH TRACKER CHECKLIST

- Physical Activity
- Sleep Tracker
- HR Monitoring
- Blood Pressure
- Blood Sugar
- Nutrition Tracker
- Weight and Body Composition
- Stress and Mood Tracker

ACTION STEPS TO A HEALTHIER YOU:

_____
_____
_____

ACCOUNTABILITY TEAM:

_____
_____
_____

Goal of the Week

To Do List:

Date _____
Month _____

SUNDAY	MONDAY	TUESDAY	WEDNESDAY	THURSDAY	FRIDAY	SATURDAY
☐	☐	☐	☐	☐	☐	☐

CREATE YOUR ENVIRONMENT/SET UP THE ATMOSPHERE:

_____
_____
_____
_____

WEEKLY REFLECTION:

- Morning Five ○○○○○○○
- HIIT Workout ○○○
- 20 Minute Walk ○○○○
- Night Cap Three ○○○○○○
- Water Goal Met ○○○○○○○

Goal of the Week

To Do List:
_____

Date _____
Month _____

☐	**SUNDAY**
☐	**MONDAY**
☐	**TUESDAY**
☐	**WEDNESDAY**
☐	**THURSDAY**
☐	**FRIDAY**
☐	**SATURDAY**

CREATE YOUR ENVIRONMENT/SET UP THE ATMOSPHERE:

WEEKLY REFLECTION:

Morning Five ○○○○○○○
HIIT Workout ○○○
20 Minute Walk ○○○○
Night Cap Three ○○○○○○
Water Goal Met ○○○○○○○

Goal of the Week

To Do List:

Date _____
Month _____

SUNDAY ☐	MONDAY ☐	TUESDAY ☐	WEDNESDAY ☐	THURSDAY ☐	FRIDAY ☐	SATURDAY ☐

CREATE YOUR ENVIRONMENT/SET UP THE ATMOSPHERE:

_____
_____
_____
_____

WEEKLY REFLECTION:

Morning Five ○○○○○○○
HIIT Workout ○○○
20 Minute Walk ○○○○
Night Cap Three ○○○○○○○
Water Goal Met ○○○○○○○

Goal of the Week

To Do List:

Date _____
Month _____

☐ SUNDAY	
☐ MONDAY	
☐ TUESDAY	
☐ WEDNESDAY	
☐ THURSDAY	
☐ FRIDAY	
☐ SATURDAY	

CREATE YOUR ENVIRONMENT/SET UP THE ATMOSPHERE:

_____
_____
_____
_____
_____
_____

WEEKLY REFLECTION:

Morning Five ○○○○○○○
HIIT Workout ○○○
20 Minute Walk ○○○○
Night Cap Three ○○○○○○
Water Goal Met ○○○○○○

Goal of the Week

To Do List:

Date _____
Month _____

SUNDAY ☐	
MONDAY ☐	
TUESDAY ☐	
WEDNESDAY ☐	
THURSDAY ☐	
FRIDAY ☐	
SATURDAY ☐	

CREATE YOUR ENVIRONMENT/SET UP THE ATMOSPHERE:

_____
_____
_____
_____

WEEKLY REFLECTION:

- Morning Five ○○○○○○
- HIIT Workout ○○○
- 20 Minute Walk ○○○○
- Night Cap Three ○○○○○○
- Water Goal Met ○○○○○○

_____
_____
_____
_____

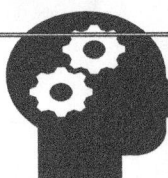

Reflection of the Month

Top 5 victories

1.
2.
3.
4.
5.

What did you learn?

1.
2.
3.
4.

List any setbacks/Obstacles

1.
2.
3.
4.
5.

What health Goals did you accomplish?

1.
2.
3.
4.
5.

What personal goals did you accomplish?

1.
2.
3.
4.
5.

What obstacles did I overcome?

1.
2.
3.
4.

What will I do differently next Month?

1.
2.
3.
4.
5

Month

Health Goal of the Month: _____

SUNDAY	MONDAY	TUESDAY	WEDNESDAY	THURSDAY	FRIDAY	SATURDAY

HEALTH TRACKER CHECKLIST

- Physical Activity
- Sleep Tracker
- HR Monitoring
- Blood Pressure
- Blood Sugar
- Nutrition Tracker
- Weight and Body Composition
- Stress and Mood Tracker

ACTION STEPS TO A HEALTHIER YOU:

ACCOUNTABILITY TEAM:

Goal of the Week

To Do List:

Date _____
Month _____

SUNDAY ☐	
MONDAY ☐	
TUESDAY ☐	
WEDNESDAY ☐	
THURSDAY ☐	
FRIDAY ☐	
SATURDAY ☐	

CREATE YOUR ENVIRONMENT/SET UP THE ATMOSPHERE:

WEEKLY REFLECTION:

- Morning Five ○○○○○○○
- HIIT Workout ○○○
- 20 Minute Walk ○○○○
- Night Cap Three ○○○○○○○
- Water Goal Met ○○○○○○○

Goal of the Week

To Do List:

Date _____
Month _____

SUNDAY ☐	MONDAY ☐	TUESDAY ☐	WEDNESDAY ☐	THURSDAY ☐	FRIDAY ☐	SATURDAY ☐

CREATE YOUR ENVIRONMENT/SET UP THE ATMOSPHERE:

_____
_____
_____

WEEKLY REFLECTION:

Morning Five	○	○	○	○	○	○
HIIT Workout	○	○	○			
20 Minute Walk	○	○	○	○		
Night Cap Three	○	○	○	○	○	○
Water Goal Met	○	○	○	○	○	○

Goal of the Week

To Do List:

Date _____
Month _____

SUNDAY	☐
MONDAY	☐
TUESDAY	☐
WEDNESDAY	☐
THURSDAY	☐
FRIDAY	☐
SATURDAY	☐

CREATE YOUR ENVIRONMENT/SET UP THE ATMOSPHERE:

WEEKLY REFLECTION:

- Morning Five ○○○○○○
- HIIT Workout ○○○
- 20 Minute Walk ○○○○
- Night Cap Three ○○○○○○
- Water Goal Met ○○○○○○

Goal of the Week

To Do List:

Date _____
Month _____

	Day
☐	SUNDAY
☐	MONDAY
☐	TUESDAY
☐	WEDNESDAY
☐	THURSDAY
☐	FRIDAY
☐	SATURDAY

CREATE YOUR ENVIRONMENT/SET UP THE ATMOSPHERE:

_____
_____
_____
_____

WEEKLY REFLECTION:

- **Morning Five** ○○○○○○○
- **HIIT Workout** ○○○
- **20 Minute Walk** ○○○○
- **Night Cap Three** ○○○○○○
- **Water Goal Met** ○○○○○○○

Goal of the Week

To Do List:
_____
| | | | | | | |

Date _____
Month _____

☐ SUNDAY	☐ MONDAY	☐ TUESDAY	☐ WEDNESDAY	☐ THURSDAY	☐ FRIDAY	☐ SATURDAY

CREATE YOUR ENVIRONMENT/SET UP THE ATMOSPHERE:
_____
_____
_____
_____

WEEKLY REFLECTION:

Morning Five   ○○○○○○○
HIIT Workout   ○○○
20 Minute Walk   ○○○○
Night Cap Three ○○○○○○
Water Goal Met   ○○○○○○○

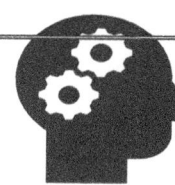

Reflection of the Month

Top 5 victories

1.
2.
3.
4.
5.

What did you learn?

1.
2.
3.
4.

List any setbacks/Obstacles

1.
2.
3.
4.
5.

What health Goals did you accomplish?

1.
2.
3.
4.
5.

What personal goals did you accomplish?

1.
2.
3.
4.
5.

What obstacles did I overcome?

1.
2.
3.
4.

What will I do differently next Month?

1.
2.
3.
4.
5.

Welcome to the "My Own PCP (Personal Care Provider)" journey, a transformative tool designed to help you take charge of your health and well-being. Created by Danielle Shears, a Registered Nurse with over 30 years of experience in multiple medical specialties, this workbook brings a fresh, holistic approach to healthcare. Drawing on Danielle's extensive background in functional nutrition and her deep understanding of the body's unique needs, this guide will empower you to move beyond symptom management and toward true healing.

In these pages, you'll discover practical tools, resources, and personalized strategies that will help you address the root causes of your health challenges, unlock your body's potential, and start feeling your best.

Meet Danielle Shears

Danielle Shears is a Registered Nurse with a wealth of experience spanning Neurology, Cardiology, Gynecology, Orthopedics, and beyond. With a Bachelor of Science in Nursing (BSN) from the University of North Carolina, an MBA in Healthcare Administration, and certifications in Neuroscience (CNRN) and Functional Nutrition (CFNC), Danielle has seen firsthand how traditional medicine often fails to address the root causes of health issues.

Driven by her passion for true healing, Danielle shifted her focus to functional nutrition, aiming to provide holistic care that empowers individuals to take control of their health. After founding **Better Choice Health LLC (BCH)**, she's been helping clients tackle chronic fatigue, autoimmunity, nutrient deficiencies, stress, and more—by offering personalized solutions that address the whole body, mind, and spirit.

Danielle's mission is simple: to help you unlock the keys to your own healing by combining nutrition, mind-body balance, and holistic wellness. With her expertise, you'll gain the tools you need to take charge of your health and truly thrive.

www.ingramcontent.com/pod-product-compliance
Lightning Source LLC
Chambersburg PA
CBHW080520030426
42337CB00023B/4573